Copyright© 2019 by Celery Juice Journals
All rights reserved. This book or any portion thereof may not be reproduced in any form in any manner whatsoever without express written permission of the publisher except for the use of brief quotations in a book review.

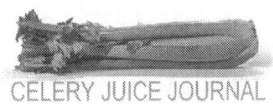

let the healing begin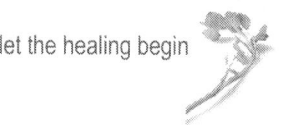

This Journal Belongs To:

_____

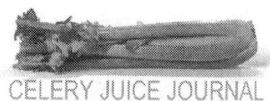
CELERY JUICE JOURNAL

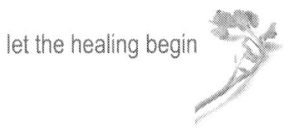

let the healing begin

Cross Out Every Day You Drink Your Celery Juice

start here

1	2	3	4	5	6	7
8	9	10	11	12	13	14
15	16	17	18	19	20	21
22	23	24	25	26	27	28
29	30	31	32	33	34	35
36	37	38	39	40	41	42
43	44	45	46	47	48	49
50	51	52	53	54	55	56
57	58	59	60	61	62	63
64	65	66	67	68	69	70
71	72	73	74	75	76	77
78	79	80	81	82	83	84
85	86	87	88	89	90	**90 Days!**

Way To Go!

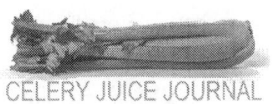

CELERY JUICE JOURNAL

let the healing begin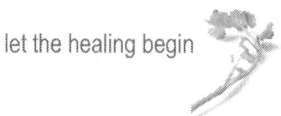

S M T W TH F S

Day # _____   Amount of Celery Juice: _____

Date: _____   Time of Celery Juice: _____

Water: ☐☐☐☐☐   How I Feel Today: _____
       ☐☐☐☐☐   _____

# Hours Sleep	Bedtime	Wake Time	Sleep Quality
			😊 🙂 😐 🙁 😵

Breakfast	Lunch	Dinner	Snacks

Notes:
_____
_____
_____
_____
_____
_____
_____
_____
_____
_____

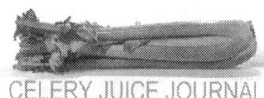
CELERY JUICE JOURNAL

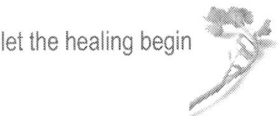

let the healing begin

S   M   T   W   TH   F   S

Day # _____

Date: _____

Water: ☐☐☐☐☐ ☐☐☐☐☐

Amount of Celery Juice: _____

Time of Celery Juice: _____

How I Feel Today: _____

# Hours Sleep	Bedtime	Wake Time	Sleep Quality ☺ ☺ ☹ ☹ ☠

Breakfast	Lunch	Dinner .	Snacks

Notes:
_____
_____
_____
_____
_____
_____
_____
_____
_____
_____

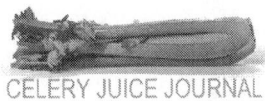

CELERY JUICE JOURNAL

let the healing begin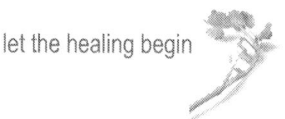

S   M   T   W   TH   F   S

Day # _____   Amount of Celery Juice: _____

Date: _____   Time of Celery Juice: _____

Water: ☐☐☐☐☐   How I Feel Today: _____
☐☐☐☐☐   _____

# Hours Sleep	Bedtime	Wake Time	Sleep Quality ☺ ☺ ☹ ☹ ☠

Breakfast	Lunch	Dinner .	Snacks

Notes:
_____
_____
_____
_____
_____
_____
_____
_____
_____

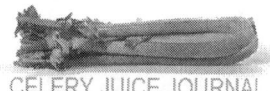
CELERY JUICE JOURNAL

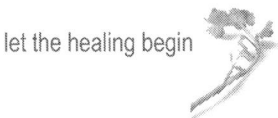

let the healing begin

S M T W TH F S

Day # _____   Amount of Celery Juice: _____

Date: _____   Time of Celery Juice: _____

Water: ☐☐☐☐☐   How I Feel Today: _____
☐☐☐☐☐   _____

# Hours Sleep	Bedtime	Wake Time	Sleep Quality
			😊 🙂 😕 ☹️ 😣

Breakfast	Lunch	Dinner	Snacks

Notes: _____
_____
_____
_____
_____
_____
_____
_____
_____
_____
_____

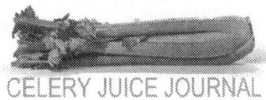

CELERY JUICE JOURNAL

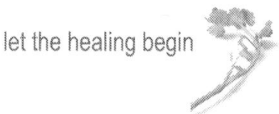
let the healing begin

S M T W TH F S

Day # _____   Amount of Celery Juice: _____

Date: _____   Time of Celery Juice: _____

Water: ☐☐☐☐☐   How I Feel Today: _____
       ☐☐☐☐☐   _____

# Hours Sleep	Bedtime	Wake Time	Sleep Quality 😊 🙂 😐 🙁 😣

Breakfast	Lunch	Dinner .	Snacks

Notes:
_____
_____
_____
_____
_____
_____
_____
_____
_____
_____

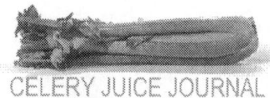
CELERY JUICE JOURNAL

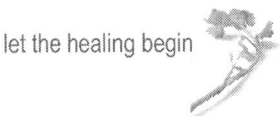

let the healing begin

S   M   T   W   TH   F   S

Day # _____   Amount of Celery Juice: _____

Date: _____   Time of Celery Juice: _____

Water: ☐☐☐☐☐   How I Feel Today: _____
       ☐☐☐☐☐   _____

# Hours Sleep	Bedtime	Wake Time	Sleep Quality
			😊 🙂 😐 ☹️ 😵

Breakfast	Lunch	Dinner	Snacks

Notes: _____
_____
_____
_____
_____
_____
_____
_____
_____
_____

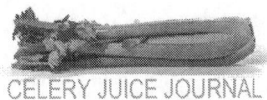

CELERY JUICE JOURNAL

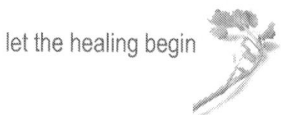

let the healing begin

S M T W TH F S

Day # _____

Date: _____

Water: ☐☐☐☐☐
☐☐☐☐☐

Amount of Celery Juice: _____

Time of Celery Juice: _____

How I Feel Today: _____
_____

# Hours Sleep	Bedtime	Wake Time	Sleep Quality ☺ ☺ ☹ ☹ ☒

Breakfast	Lunch	Dinner .	Snacks

Notes:
_____
_____
_____
_____
_____
_____
_____
_____
_____

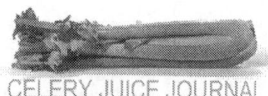

CELERY JUICE JOURNAL

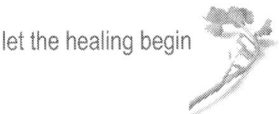
let the healing begin

S M T W TH F S

Day # _____   Amount of Celery Juice: _____

Date: _____   Time of Celery Juice: _____

Water: ☐☐☐☐☐   How I Feel Today: _____
       ☐☐☐☐☐   _____

# Hours Sleep	Bedtime	Wake Time	Sleep Quality ☺ ☺ ☹ ☹ ☠

Breakfast	Lunch	Dinner	Snacks

Notes:
_____
_____
_____
_____
_____
_____
_____
_____
_____
_____

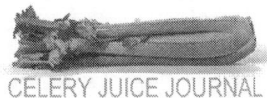
CELERY JUICE JOURNAL

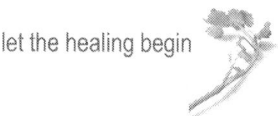

let the healing begin

S M T W TH F S

Day # _____

Date: _____

Water: ☐☐☐☐☐
☐☐☐☐☐

Amount of Celery Juice: _____

Time of Celery Juice: _____

How I Feel Today: _____
_____

# Hours Sleep	Bedtime	Wake Time	Sleep Quality 😊 🙂 😐 🙁 😣

Breakfast	Lunch	Dinner .	Snacks

Notes:
_____
_____
_____
_____
_____
_____
_____
_____
_____
_____
_____

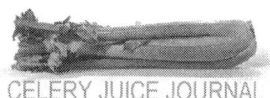

CELERY JUICE JOURNAL

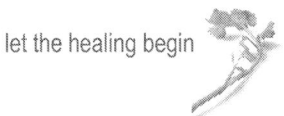
let the healing begin

S   M   T   W   TH   F   S

Day # _____   Amount of Celery Juice: _____

Date: _____   Time of Celery Juice: _____

Water: ☐☐☐☐☐   How I Feel Today: _____
       ☐☐☐☐☐   _____

# Hours Sleep	Bedtime	Wake Time	Sleep Quality
			😊 🙂 😐 ☹ 😵

Breakfast	Lunch	Dinner	Snacks

Notes:
_____
_____
_____
_____
_____
_____
_____
_____
_____
_____

CELERY JUICE JOURNAL

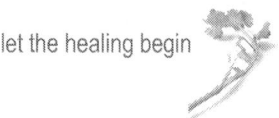
let the healing begin

S M T W TH F S

Day # _____

Date: _____

Water: ☐☐☐☐☐
       ☐☐☐☐☐

Amount of Celery Juice: _____

Time of Celery Juice: _____

How I Feel Today: _____
_____

# Hours Sleep	Bedtime	Wake Time	Sleep Quality 😊 🙂 😐 ☹️ 😖

Breakfast	Lunch	Dinner .	Snacks

Notes:
_____
_____
_____
_____
_____
_____
_____
_____
_____
_____

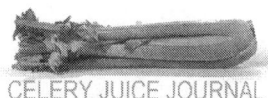
CELERY JUICE JOURNAL

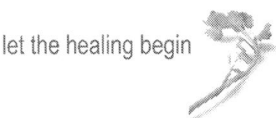
let the healing begin

S M T W TH F S

Day # _____

Date: _____

Water: ☐☐☐☐☐
☐☐☐☐☐

Amount of Celery Juice: _____

Time of Celery Juice: _____

How I Feel Today: _____
_____

# Hours Sleep	Bedtime	Wake Time	Sleep Quality 😊 🙂 😐 ☹️ 😵

Breakfast	Lunch	Dinner .	Snacks

Notes:
_____
_____
_____
_____
_____
_____
_____
_____
_____

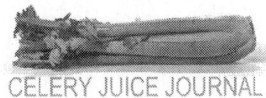
CELERY JUICE JOURNAL

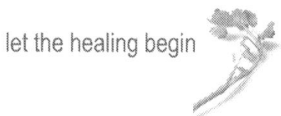

let the healing begin

S   M   T   W   TH   F   S

Day # _____   Amount of Celery Juice: _____

Date: _____   Time of Celery Juice: _____

Water: ☐☐☐☐☐   How I Feel Today: _____
☐☐☐☐☐   _____

# Hours Sleep	Bedtime	Wake Time	Sleep Quality 🙂 😐 😕 ☹ 😵

Breakfast	Lunch	Dinner	Snacks

Notes:
_____
_____
_____
_____
_____
_____
_____
_____
_____
_____
_____

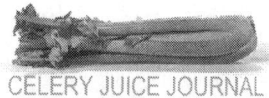

CELERY JUICE JOURNAL

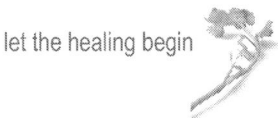
let the healing begin

S M T W TH F S

Day # _____   Amount of Celery Juice: _____

Date: _____   Time of Celery Juice: _____

Water: ⬜⬜⬜⬜⬜   How I Feel Today: _____
       ⬜⬜⬜⬜⬜   _____

# Hours Sleep	Bedtime	Wake Time	Sleep Quality
			😊 🙂 😐 ☹️ 😵

Breakfast	Lunch	Dinner	Snacks

Notes:
_____
_____
_____
_____
_____
_____
_____
_____
_____
_____

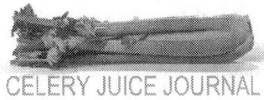
CELERY JUICE JOURNAL

let the healing begin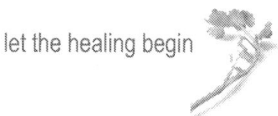

S   M   T   W   TH   F   S

Day # _____   Amount of Celery Juice: _____

Date: _____   Time of Celery Juice: _____

Water: ☐☐☐☐☐   How I Feel Today: _____
☐☐☐☐☐   _____

# Hours Sleep	Bedtime	Wake Time	Sleep Quality ☺ ☺ ☹ ☹ ☠

Breakfast	Lunch	Dinner .	Snacks

Notes: _____
_____
_____
_____
_____
_____
_____
_____
_____
_____
_____

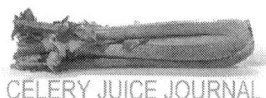
CELERY JUICE JOURNAL

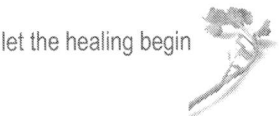

let the healing begin

S M T W TH F S

Day # _____   Amount of Celery Juice: _____

Date: _____   Time of Celery Juice: _____

Water: ☐☐☐☐☐   How I Feel Today: _____
       ☐☐☐☐☐   _____

# Hours Sleep	Bedtime	Wake Time	Sleep Quality 😊 🙂 😕 ☹️ 😵

Breakfast	Lunch	Dinner	Snacks

Notes:
_____
_____
_____
_____
_____
_____
_____
_____
_____
_____

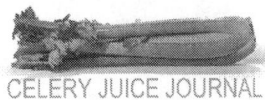

CELERY JUICE JOURNAL

let the healing begin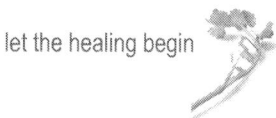

S   M   T   W   TH   F   S

Day # _____   Amount of Celery Juice: _____

Date: _____   Time of Celery Juice: _____

Water: ☐☐☐☐☐   How I Feel Today: _____
☐☐☐☐☐   _____

# Hours Sleep	Bedtime	Wake Time	Sleep Quality 😊 😐 😕 ☹ 😖

Breakfast	Lunch	Dinner .	Snacks

Notes: _____
_____
_____
_____
_____
_____
_____
_____
_____

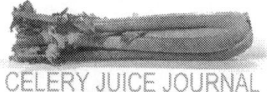
CELERY JUICE JOURNAL

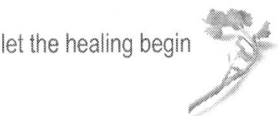
let the healing begin

S M T W TH F S

Day # _____   Amount of Celery Juice: _____

Date: _____   Time of Celery Juice: _____

Water: ☐☐☐☐☐   How I Feel Today: _____
       ☐☐☐☐☐   _____

# Hours Sleep	Bedtime	Wake Time	Sleep Quality
			😊 😐 😕 ☹️ 😵

Breakfast	Lunch	Dinner	Snacks

Notes:
_____
_____
_____
_____
_____
_____
_____
_____
_____

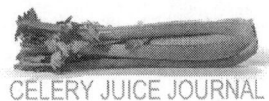
CELERY JUICE JOURNAL

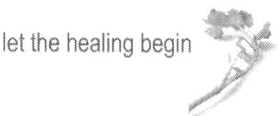
let the healing begin

S M T W TH F S

Day # _____   Amount of Celery Juice: _____

Date: _____   Time of Celery Juice: _____

Water: ☐☐☐☐☐   How I Feel Today: _____
       ☐☐☐☐☐   _____

# Hours Sleep	Bedtime	Wake Time	Sleep Quality 😊 🙂 😐 ☹️ 😵

Breakfast	Lunch	Dinner .	Snacks

Notes:
_____
_____
_____
_____
_____
_____
_____
_____
_____

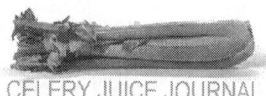
CELERY JUICE JOURNAL

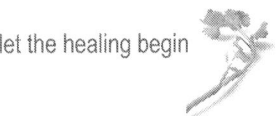

let the healing begin

S M T W TH F S

Day #: _____

Date: _____

Water: ☐ ☐ ☐ ☐ ☐ ☐ ☐ ☐ ☐ ☐

Amount of Celery Juice: _____

Time of Celery Juice: _____

How I Feel Today: _____

# Hours Sleep	Bedtime	Wake Time	Sleep Quality
			😊 🙂 😐 😦 😵

Breakfast	Lunch	Dinner	Snacks

Notes: _____

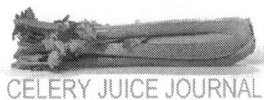

CELERY JUICE JOURNAL

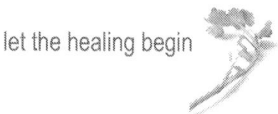
let the healing begin

S   M   T   W   TH   F   S

Day # _____   Amount of Celery Juice: _____

Date: _____   Time of Celery Juice: _____

Water: ☐☐☐☐☐   How I Feel Today: _____
       ☐☐☐☐☐   _____

# Hours Sleep	Bedtime	Wake Time	Sleep Quality 😊 🙂 😐 🙁 😵

Breakfast	Lunch	Dinner	Snacks

Notes:
_____
_____
_____
_____
_____
_____
_____
_____
_____

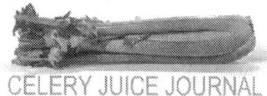
CELERY JUICE JOURNAL

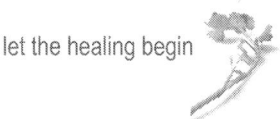

let the healing begin

S   M   T   W   TH   F   S

Day # _____

Date: _____

Water: ☐☐☐☐☐
       ☐☐☐☐☐

Amount of Celery Juice: _____

Time of Celery Juice: _____

How I Feel Today: _____
_____

# Hours Sleep	Bedtime	Wake Time	Sleep Quality 😊 🙂 😐 ☹️ 😵

Breakfast	Lunch	Dinner	Snacks

Notes:
_____
_____
_____
_____
_____
_____
_____
_____
_____

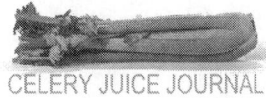

CELERY JUICE JOURNAL

let the healing begin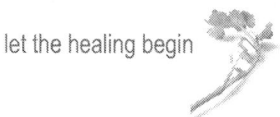

S M T W TH F S

Day # _____   Amount of Celery Juice: _____

Date: _____   Time of Celery Juice: _____

Water: ☐☐☐☐☐   How I Feel Today: _____
☐☐☐☐☐   _____

# Hours Sleep	Bedtime	Wake Time	Sleep Quality
			😊 🙂 😐 🙁 😵

Breakfast	Lunch	Dinner .	Snacks

Notes:
_____
_____
_____
_____
_____
_____
_____
_____
_____
_____
_____

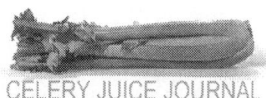
CELERY JUICE JOURNAL

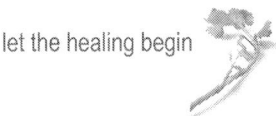
let the healing begin

S M T W TH F S

Day # _____

Date: _____

Water: ☐☐☐☐☐
       ☐☐☐☐☐

Amount of Celery Juice: _____

Time of Celery Juice: _____

How I Feel Today: _____
_____

# Hours Sleep	Bedtime	Wake Time	Sleep Quality 😊 🙂 😐 😟 😵

Breakfast	Lunch	Dinner .	Snacks

Notes:
_____
_____
_____
_____
_____
_____
_____
_____
_____

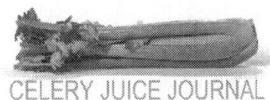
CELERY JUICE JOURNAL

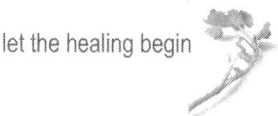
let the healing begin

S M T W TH F S

Day # _____

Date: _____

Water: ☐ ☐ ☐ ☐ ☐
☐ ☐ ☐ ☐ ☐

Amount of Celery Juice: _____

Time of Celery Juice: _____

How I Feel Today: _____
_____

# Hours Sleep	Bedtime	Wake Time	Sleep Quality 😊 🙂 😐 🙁 😵

Breakfast	Lunch	Dinner .	Snacks

Notes:
_____
_____
_____
_____
_____
_____
_____
_____
_____
_____

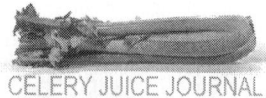
CELERY JUICE JOURNAL

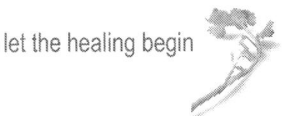

let the healing begin

S M T W TH F S

Day # _____   Amount of Celery Juice: _____

Date: _____   Time of Celery Juice: _____

Water: ☐☐☐☐☐   How I Feel Today: _____
       ☐☐☐☐☐   _____

# Hours Sleep	Bedtime	Wake Time	Sleep Quality
			😊 😐 😕 ☹️ ✖✖

Breakfast	Lunch	Dinner	Snacks

Notes: _____
_____
_____
_____
_____
_____
_____
_____
_____
_____

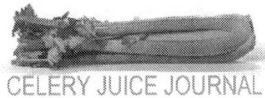

CELERY JUICE JOURNAL

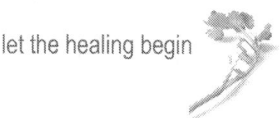
let the healing begin

S M T W TH F S

Day # _____   Amount of Celery Juice: _____

Date: _____   Time of Celery Juice: _____

Water: ☐☐☐☐☐   How I Feel Today: _____
       ☐☐☐☐☐   _____

# Hours Sleep	Bedtime	Wake Time	Sleep Quality 😊 🙂 😐 ☹️ 😵

Breakfast	Lunch	Dinner .	Snacks

Notes:
_____
_____
_____
_____
_____
_____
_____
_____
_____
_____

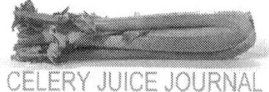
CELERY JUICE JOURNAL

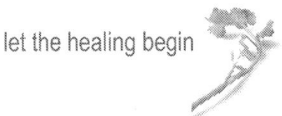

let the healing begin

S M T W TH F S

Day # _____

Date: _____

Water: ☐☐☐☐☐
☐☐☐☐☐

Amount of Celery Juice: _____

Time of Celery Juice: _____

How I Feel Today: _____
_____

# Hours Sleep	Bedtime	Wake Time	Sleep Quality 😊 🙂 😐 😕 😵

Breakfast	Lunch	Dinner .	Snacks

Notes: _____
_____
_____
_____
_____
_____
_____
_____
_____
_____

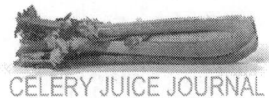

CELERY JUICE JOURNAL

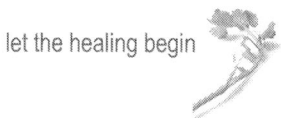
let the healing begin

S M T W TH F S

Day # _____   Amount of Celery Juice: _____

Date: _____   Time of Celery Juice: _____

Water: ☐☐☐☐☐   How I Feel Today: _____
☐☐☐☐☐   _____

# Hours Sleep	Bedtime	Wake Time	Sleep Quality 😊 🙂 😐 🙁 😵

Breakfast	Lunch	Dinner	Snacks

Notes:
_____
_____
_____
_____
_____
_____
_____
_____
_____

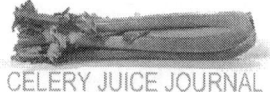
CELERY JUICE JOURNAL

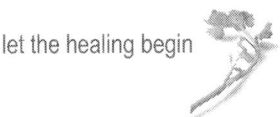
let the healing begin

S M T W TH F S

Day # _____   Amount of Celery Juice: _____

Date: _____   Time of Celery Juice: _____

Water: ☐☐☐☐☐   How I Feel Today: _____
       ☐☐☐☐☐   _____

# Hours Sleep	Bedtime	Wake Time	Sleep Quality 😊 🙂 😐 🙁 😵

Breakfast	Lunch	Dinner .	Snacks

Notes:
_____
_____
_____
_____
_____
_____
_____
_____
_____

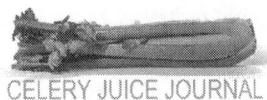
CELERY JUICE JOURNAL

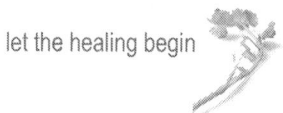

let the healing begin

S   M   T   W   TH   F   S

Day # _____   Amount of Celery Juice: _____

Date: _____   Time of Celery Juice: _____

Water: ☐☐☐☐☐   How I Feel Today: _____
       ☐☐☐☐☐   _____

# Hours Sleep	Bedtime	Wake Time	Sleep Quality 😊 🙂 😐 🙁 😵

Breakfast	Lunch	Dinner .	Snacks

Notes:
_____
_____
_____
_____
_____
_____
_____
_____
_____
_____

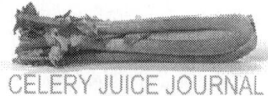

CELERY JUICE JOURNAL

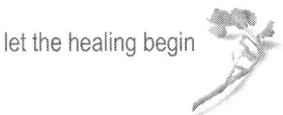
let the healing begin

S M T W TH F S

Day # _____   Amount of Celery Juice: _____

Date: _____   Time of Celery Juice: _____

Water: ☐☐☐☐☐   How I Feel Today: _____
       ☐☐☐☐☐   _____

# Hours Sleep	Bedtime	Wake Time	Sleep Quality
			😊 🙂 😐 ☹ 😵

Breakfast	Lunch	Dinner .	Snacks

Notes: _____
_____
_____
_____
_____
_____
_____
_____
_____
_____

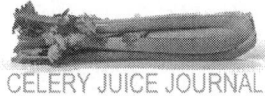
CELERY JUICE JOURNAL

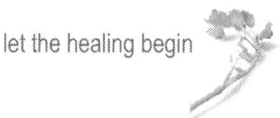

let the healing begin

S M T W TH F S

Day # _____   Amount of Celery Juice: _____

Date: _____   Time of Celery Juice: _____

Water: ☐☐☐☐☐   How I Feel Today: _____
☐☐☐☐☐   _____

# Hours Sleep	Bedtime	Wake Time	Sleep Quality 😊😃😐☹😵

Breakfast	Lunch	Dinner .	Snacks

Notes:
_____
_____
_____
_____
_____
_____
_____
_____
_____

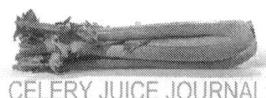

CELERY JUICE JOURNAL

let the healing begin

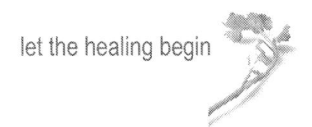

S   M   T   W   TH   F   S

Day # _____   Amount of Celery Juice: _____

Date: _____   Time of Celery Juice: _____

Water: ☐☐☐☐☐   How I Feel Today: _____
       ☐☐☐☐☐   _____

# Hours Sleep	Bedtime	Wake Time	Sleep Quality
			😊 🙂 😐 ☹️ 😵

Breakfast	Lunch	Dinner	Snacks

Notes: _____
_____
_____
_____
_____
_____
_____
_____
_____

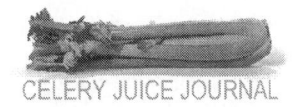

CELERY JUICE JOURNAL

let the healing begin

S M T W TH F S

Day # _____

Date: _____

Water: ☐☐☐☐☐ ☐☐☐☐☐

Amount of Celery Juice: _____

Time of Celery Juice: _____

How I Feel Today: _____
_____

# Hours Sleep	Bedtime	Wake Time	Sleep Quality 😊 🙂 😐 🙁 😣

Breakfast	Lunch	Dinner	Snacks

Notes:
_____
_____
_____
_____
_____
_____
_____
_____
_____
_____

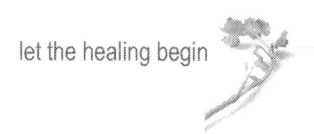

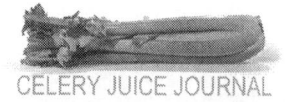

CELERY JUICE JOURNAL

let the healing begin

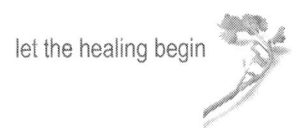

S M T W TH F S

Day # _____

Date: _____

Water: ☐☐☐☐☐ ☐☐☐☐☐

Amount of Celery Juice: _____

Time of Celery Juice: _____

How I Feel Today: _____
_____

# Hours Sleep	Bedtime	Wake Time	Sleep Quality 😊 ☺ 😐 ☹ 😵

Breakfast	Lunch	Dinner .	Snacks

Notes: _____
_____
_____
_____
_____
_____
_____
_____
_____
_____

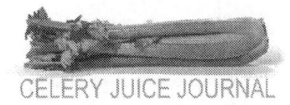

CELERY JUICE JOURNAL

let the healing begin

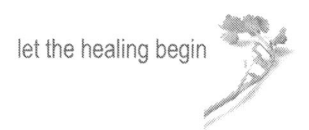

S   M   T   W   TH   F   S

Day # _____   Amount of Celery Juice: _____

Date: _____   Time of Celery Juice: _____

Water: ☐☐☐☐☐   How I Feel Today: _____
       ☐☐☐☐☐   _____

# Hours Sleep	Bedtime	Wake Time	Sleep Quality
			😊 🙂 😐 ☹️ 😵

Breakfast	Lunch	Dinner .	Snacks

Notes: _____
_____
_____
_____
_____
_____
_____
_____
_____
_____

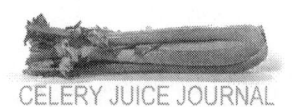

CELERY JUICE JOURNAL

let the healing begin

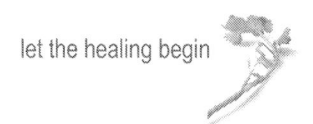

S M T W TH F S

Day # _____ Amount of Celery Juice: _____

Date: _____ Time of Celery Juice: _____

Water: ☐☐☐☐☐☐ How I Feel Today: _____
       ☐☐☐☐☐☐   _____

# Hours Sleep	Bedtime	Wake Time	Sleep Quality
			😊 🙂 😐 ☹️ 😵

Breakfast	Lunch	Dinner	Snacks

Notes: _____
_____
_____
_____
_____
_____
_____
_____
_____
_____

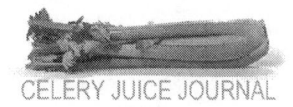

CELERY JUICE JOURNAL

let the healing begin

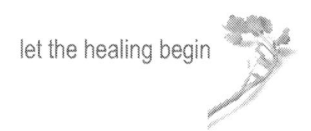

S M T W TH F S

Day # _____

Date: _____

Water: ☐☐☐☐☐
☐☐☐☐☐

Amount of Celery Juice: _____

Time of Celery Juice: _____

How I Feel Today: _____
_____

# Hours Sleep	Bedtime	Wake Time	Sleep Quality 😊 🙂 😐 🙁 😵

Breakfast	Lunch	Dinner .	Snacks

Notes:
_____
_____
_____
_____
_____
_____
_____
_____
_____
_____

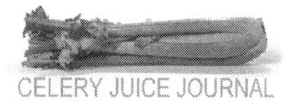

CELERY JUICE JOURNAL

let the healing begin

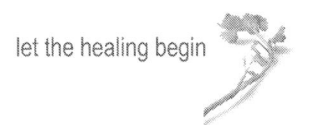

S   M   T   W   TH   F   S

Day # _____

Date: _____

Water: ☐ ☐ ☐ ☐ ☐
☐ ☐ ☐ ☐ ☐

Amount of Celery Juice: _____

Time of Celery Juice: _____

How I Feel Today: _____
_____

# Hours Sleep	Bedtime	Wake Time	Sleep Quality
			😊 🙂 😐 ☹️ 😵

Breakfast	Lunch	Dinner	Snacks

Notes:
_____
_____
_____
_____
_____
_____
_____
_____
_____
_____

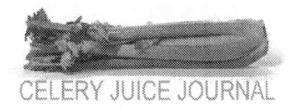

CELERY JUICE JOURNAL

let the healing begin

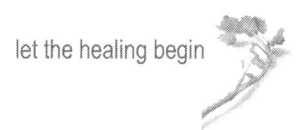

S M T W TH F S

Day # _____   Amount of Celery Juice: _____

Date: _____   Time of Celery Juice: _____

Water: ☐☐☐☐☐   How I Feel Today: _____
       ☐☐☐☐☐   _____

# Hours Sleep	Bedtime	Wake Time	Sleep Quality 😊 🙂 😐 😕 😫

Breakfast	Lunch	Dinner	Snacks

Notes:
_____
_____
_____
_____
_____
_____
_____
_____
_____
_____

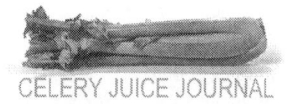

CELERY JUICE JOURNAL

let the healing begin

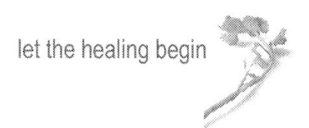

S M T W TH F S

Day # _____

Date: _____

Water: ☐☐☐☐☐
☐☐☐☐☐

Amount of Celery Juice: _____

Time of Celery Juice: _____

How I Feel Today: _____
_____

# Hours Sleep	Bedtime	Wake Time	Sleep Quality
			😊 🙂 😐 ☹️ 😵

Breakfast	Lunch	Dinner .	Snacks

Notes:
_____
_____
_____
_____
_____
_____
_____
_____
_____
_____

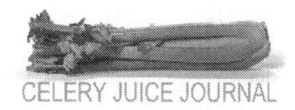

CELERY JUICE JOURNAL

let the healing begin

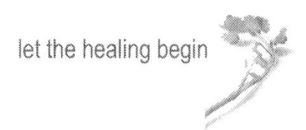

S M T W TH F S

Day # _____

Date: _____

Water: ☐☐☐☐☐
       ☐☐☐☐☐

Amount of Celery Juice: _____

Time of Celery Juice: _____

How I Feel Today: _____
_____

# Hours Sleep	Bedtime	Wake Time	Sleep Quality 😊 🙂 😐 🙁 😵

Breakfast	Lunch	Dinner .	Snacks

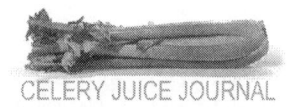

Notes:
_____
_____
_____
_____
_____
_____
_____
_____
_____
_____

CELERY JUICE JOURNAL

let the healing begin

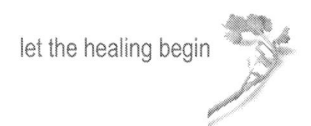

S M T W TH F S

Day # _____   Amount of Celery Juice: _____

Date: _____   Time of Celery Juice: _____

Water: ☐☐☐☐☐   How I Feel Today: _____
☐☐☐☐☐   _____

# Hours Sleep	Bedtime	Wake Time	Sleep Quality
			😊 🙂 😐 ☹️ 😵

Breakfast	Lunch	Dinner .	Snacks

Notes:
_____
_____
_____
_____
_____
_____
_____
_____
_____
_____

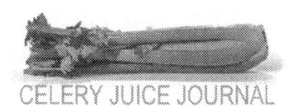

CELERY JUICE JOURNAL

let the healing begin

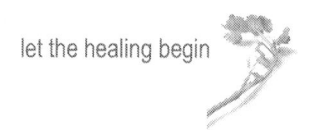

S   M   T   W   TH   F   S

Day # _____

Date: _____

Water: ☐☐☐☐☐
☐☐☐☐☐

Amount of Celery Juice: _____

Time of Celery Juice: _____

How I Feel Today: _____
_____

# Hours Sleep	Bedtime	Wake Time	Sleep Quality 😊 🙂 😐 ☹️ 😵

Breakfast	Lunch	Dinner .	Snacks

Notes:
_____
_____
_____
_____
_____
_____
_____
_____
_____
_____

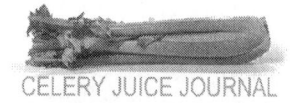

CELERY JUICE JOURNAL

let the healing begin

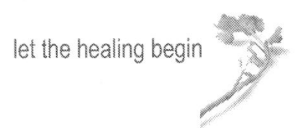

S   M   T   W   TH   F   S

Day # _____

Date: _____

Water: ☐☐☐☐☐
☐☐☐☐☐

Amount of Celery Juice: _____

Time of Celery Juice: _____

How I Feel Today: _____
_____

# Hours Sleep	Bedtime	Wake Time	Sleep Quality
			😊 🙂 😐 😟 😫

Breakfast	Lunch	Dinner	Snacks

Notes:
_____
_____
_____
_____
_____
_____
_____
_____
_____
_____

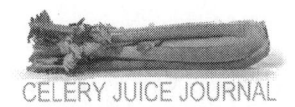

CELERY JUICE JOURNAL

let the healing begin

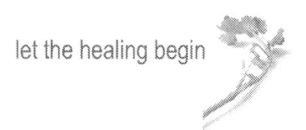

S M T W TH F S

Day # _____   Amount of Celery Juice: _____

Date: _____   Time of Celery Juice: _____

Water: ☐☐☐☐☐   How I Feel Today: _____
       ☐☐☐☐☐   _____

# Hours Sleep	Bedtime	Wake Time	Sleep Quality
			😊 😐 😕 ☹️ 😣

Breakfast	Lunch	Dinner .	Snacks

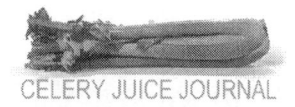

Notes: _____
_____
_____
_____
_____
_____
_____
_____
_____
_____

CELERY JUICE JOURNAL

let the healing begin

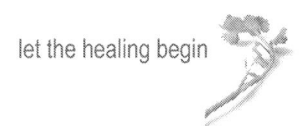

S   M   T   W   TH   F   S

Day # _____

Date: _____

Water: ☐☐☐☐☐
       ☐☐☐☐☐

Amount of Celery Juice: _____

Time of Celery Juice: _____

How I Feel Today: _____
_____

# Hours Sleep	Bedtime	Wake Time	Sleep Quality 😊😃😐😕😖

Breakfast	Lunch	Dinner .	Snacks

Notes:
_____
_____
_____
_____
_____
_____
_____
_____
_____

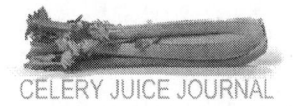

CELERY JUICE JOURNAL

let the healing begin

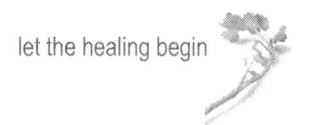

S M T W TH F S

Day # _____   Amount of Celery Juice: _____

Date: _____   Time of Celery Juice: _____

Water: ☐☐☐☐☐   How I Feel Today: _____
       ☐☐☐☐☐   _____

# Hours Sleep	Bedtime	Wake Time	Sleep Quality
			😊 😐 😕 😟 😵

Breakfast	Lunch	Dinner	Snacks

Notes: _____

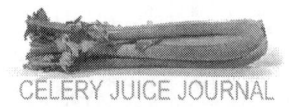

_____

_____

_____

_____

_____

_____

_____

_____

_____

_____

CELERY JUICE JOURNAL

let the healing begin

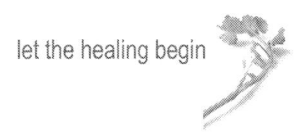

S M T W TH F S

Day # _____

Date: _____

Water: ▢▢▢▢▢
▢▢▢▢▢

Amount of Celery Juice: _____

Time of Celery Juice: _____

How I Feel Today: _____
_____

# Hours Sleep	Bedtime	Wake Time	Sleep Quality 😊 🙂 😐 🙁 😵

Breakfast	Lunch	Dinner.	Snacks

Notes:
_____
_____
_____
_____
_____
_____
_____
_____
_____
_____

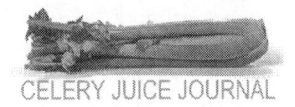

CELERY JUICE JOURNAL

let the healing begin

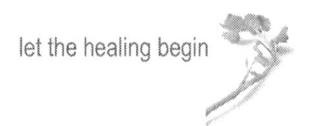

S M T W TH F S

Day # _____   Amount of Celery Juice: _____

Date: _____   Time of Celery Juice: _____

Water: ☐☐☐☐☐   How I Feel Today: _____
       ☐☐☐☐☐   _____

# Hours Sleep	Bedtime	Wake Time	Sleep Quality
			😊 🙂 😐 😟 😣

Breakfast	Lunch	Dinner .	Snacks

Notes:
_____
_____
_____
_____
_____
_____
_____
_____
_____
_____

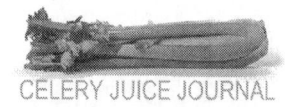

CELERY JUICE JOURNAL

let the healing begin

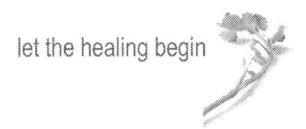

S M T W TH F S

Day # _____

Date: _____

Water: ☐☐☐☐☐
☐☐☐☐☐

Amount of Celery Juice: _____

Time of Celery Juice: _____

How I Feel Today: _____
_____

# Hours Sleep	Bedtime	Wake Time	Sleep Quality 😊 🙂 😐 ☹️ 😣

Breakfast	Lunch	Dinner	Snacks

Notes:
_____
_____
_____
_____
_____
_____
_____
_____
_____
_____
_____

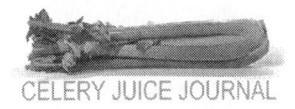

CELERY JUICE JOURNAL

let the healing begin

S M T W TH F S

Day # _____

Date: _____

Water: ☐☐☐☐☐ ☐☐☐☐☐

Amount of Celery Juice: _____

Time of Celery Juice: _____

How I Feel Today: _____

# Hours Sleep	Bedtime	Wake Time	Sleep Quality
			😊 😃 😐 😟 😵

Breakfast	Lunch	Dinner	Snacks

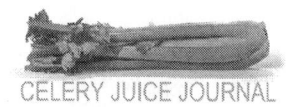

Notes: _____

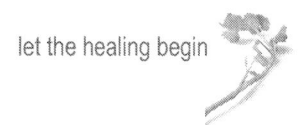

_____

_____

_____

_____

_____

_____

_____

_____

_____

CELERY JUICE JOURNAL

let the healing begin

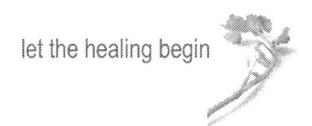

S M T W TH F S

Day # _____

Date: _____

Water: ☐☐☐☐☐
       ☐☐☐☐☐

Amount of Celery Juice: _____

Time of Celery Juice: _____

How I Feel Today: _____
_____

# Hours Sleep	Bedtime	Wake Time	Sleep Quality 😊 🙂 😐 🙁 😫

Breakfast	Lunch	Dinner .	Snacks

Notes:
_____
_____
_____
_____
_____
_____
_____
_____
_____
_____

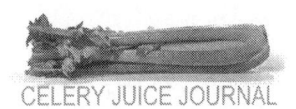

CELERY JUICE JOURNAL

let the healing begin

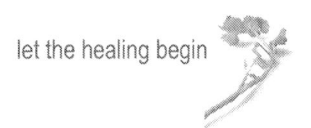

S M T W TH F S

Day # _____

Date: _____

Water: ☐☐☐☐☐
       ☐☐☐☐☐

Amount of Celery Juice: _____

Time of Celery Juice: _____

How I Feel Today: _____
_____

# Hours Sleep	Bedtime	Wake Time	Sleep Quality 😊 😉 😐 😟 😵

Breakfast	Lunch	Dinner .	Snacks

Notes:
_____
_____
_____
_____
_____
_____
_____
_____
_____
_____

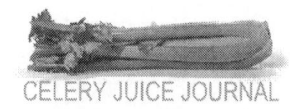

CELERY JUICE JOURNAL

let the healing begin

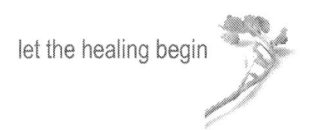

S M T W TH F S

Day # _____   Amount of Celery Juice: _____

Date: _____   Time of Celery Juice: _____

Water: ☐☐☐☐☐   How I Feel Today: _____
       ☐☐☐☐☐   _____

# Hours Sleep	Bedtime	Wake Time	Sleep Quality 😊 🙂 😐 ☹️ 😣

Breakfast	Lunch	Dinner	Snacks

Notes:
_____
_____
_____
_____
_____
_____
_____
_____
_____
_____
_____

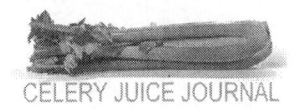

CELERY JUICE JOURNAL

let the healing begin

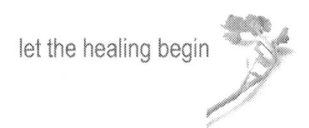

S   M   T   W   TH   F   S

Day # _____   Amount of Celery Juice: _____

Date: _____   Time of Celery Juice: _____

Water: ☐☐☐☐☐   How I Feel Today: _____
       ☐☐☐☐☐   _____

# Hours Sleep	Bedtime	Wake Time	Sleep Quality
			😊 🙂 😐 😟 😵

Breakfast	Lunch	Dinner	Snacks

Notes: _____
_____
_____
_____
_____
_____
_____
_____
_____
_____

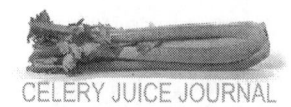

CELERY JUICE JOURNAL

let the healing begin

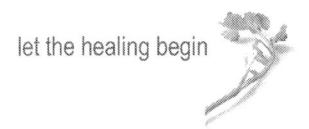

S M T W TH F S

Day # _____   Amount of Celery Juice: _____

Date: _____   Time of Celery Juice: _____

Water: ☐☐☐☐☐   How I Feel Today: _____
       ☐☐☐☐☐   _____

# Hours Sleep	Bedtime	Wake Time	Sleep Quality
			😊 🙂 😐 🙁 😵

Breakfast	Lunch	Dinner	Snacks

Notes: _____
_____
_____
_____
_____
_____
_____
_____
_____
_____
_____

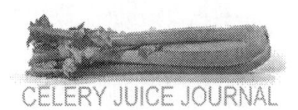

CELERY JUICE JOURNAL

let the healing begin

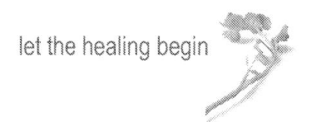

S M T W TH F S

Day # _____   Amount of Celery Juice: _____

Date: _____   Time of Celery Juice: _____

Water: ▢▢▢▢▢   How I Feel Today: _____
▢▢▢▢▢   _____

# Hours Sleep	Bedtime	Wake Time	Sleep Quality
			☺ 🙂 😐 ☹ 😫

Breakfast	Lunch	Dinner .	Snacks

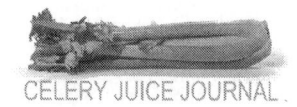

Notes: _____

_____

_____

_____

_____

_____

_____

_____

_____

_____

_____

CELERY JUICE JOURNAL

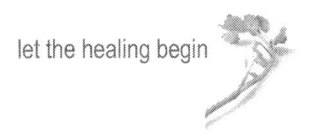

let the healing begin

S M T W TH F S

Day # _____

Date: _____

Water: ☐☐☐☐☐
☐☐☐☐☐

Amount of Celery Juice: _____

Time of Celery Juice: _____

How I Feel Today: _____
_____

# Hours Sleep	Bedtime	Wake Time	Sleep Quality
			😊 🙂 😕 🙁 😵

Breakfast	Lunch	Dinner .	Snacks

Notes: _____
_____
_____
_____
_____
_____
_____
_____
_____
_____

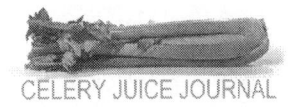

CELERY JUICE JOURNAL

let the healing begin

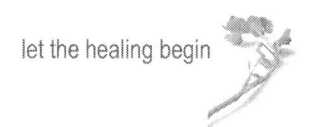

S M T W TH F S

Day # _____   Amount of Celery Juice: _____

Date: _____   Time of Celery Juice: _____

Water: ☐☐☐☐☐   How I Feel Today: _____
       ☐☐☐☐☐   _____

# Hours Sleep	Bedtime	Wake Time	Sleep Quality
			😊 🙂 😐 😟 😵

Breakfast	Lunch	Dinner .	Snacks

Notes:
_____
_____
_____
_____
_____
_____
_____
_____
_____
_____

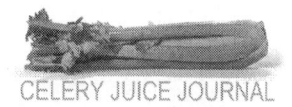

CELERY JUICE JOURNAL

let the healing begin

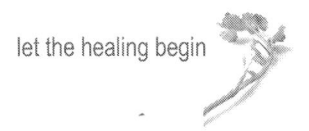

S   M   T   W   TH   F   S

Day # _____

Date: _____

Water: ☐☐☐☐☐ ☐☐☐☐☐

Amount of Celery Juice: _____

Time of Celery Juice: _____

How I Feel Today: _____
_____

# Hours Sleep	Bedtime	Wake Time	Sleep Quality
			😊 🙂 😐 ☹️ 😣

Breakfast	Lunch	Dinner .	Snacks

Notes:
_____
_____
_____
_____
_____
_____
_____
_____
_____
_____

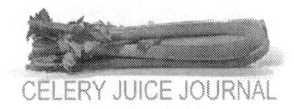

CELERY JUICE JOURNAL

let the healing begin

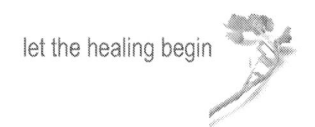

S M T W TH F S

Day # _____

Date: _____

Water: ☐☐☐☐☐
       ☐☐☐☐☐

Amount of Celery Juice: _____

Time of Celery Juice: _____

How I Feel Today: _____
_____

# Hours Sleep	Bedtime	Wake Time	Sleep Quality
			😊 🙂 😐 ☹️ 😵

Breakfast	Lunch	Dinner .	Snacks

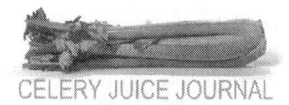

Notes:
_____
_____
_____
_____
_____
_____
_____
_____
_____
_____

CELERY JUICE JOURNAL

let the healing begin

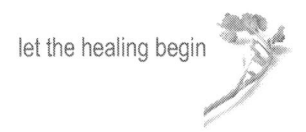

S M T W TH F S

Day # _____   Amount of Celery Juice: _____

Date: _____   Time of Celery Juice: _____

Water: ▯▯▯▯▯   How I Feel Today: _____
▯▯▯▯▯   _____

# Hours Sleep	Bedtime	Wake Time	Sleep Quality
			😊 🙂 😐 ☹️ 😵

Breakfast	Lunch	Dinner .	Snacks

Notes:
_____
_____
_____
_____
_____
_____
_____
_____
_____
_____

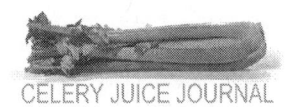

CELERY JUICE JOURNAL

let the healing begin

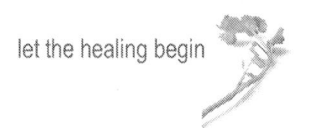

S M T W TH F S

Day # _____

Date: _____

Water: ☐☐☐☐☐
       ☐☐☐☐☐

Amount of Celery Juice: _____

Time of Celery Juice: _____

How I Feel Today: _____
_____

# Hours Sleep	Bedtime	Wake Time	Sleep Quality
			😊 🙂 😐 😟 😵

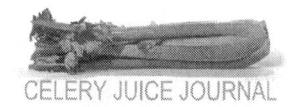

Breakfast	Lunch	Dinner .	Snacks

Notes:
_____
_____
_____
_____
_____
_____
_____
_____
_____
_____

CELERY JUICE JOURNAL

let the healing begin

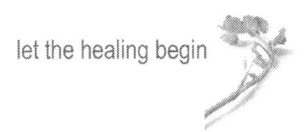

S M T W TH F S

Day # _____   Amount of Celery Juice: _____

Date: _____   Time of Celery Juice: _____

Water: ☐☐☐☐☐   How I Feel Today: _____
       ☐☐☐☐☐   _____

# Hours Sleep	Bedtime	Wake Time	Sleep Quality 😊 🙂 😕 🙁 😵

Breakfast	Lunch	Dinner .	Snacks

Notes: _____
_____
_____
_____
_____
_____
_____
_____
_____
_____

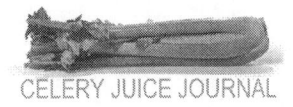

CELERY JUICE JOURNAL

let the healing begin

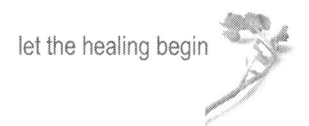

S M T W TH F S

Day # _____   Amount of Celery Juice: _____

Date: _____   Time of Celery Juice: _____

Water: ☐☐☐☐☐   How I Feel Today: _____
☐☐☐☐☐   _____

# Hours Sleep	Bedtime	Wake Time	Sleep Quality 😊😃😐😕😣

Breakfast	Lunch	Dinner .	Snacks

Notes:
_____
_____
_____
_____
_____
_____
_____
_____
_____

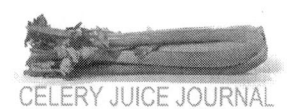

CELERY JUICE JOURNAL

let the healing begin

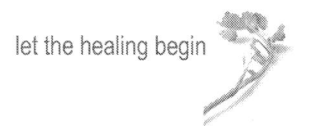

S M T W TH F S

Day # _____   Amount of Celery Juice: _____

Date: _____   Time of Celery Juice: _____

Water: ☐☐☐☐☐   How I Feel Today: _____
       ☐☐☐☐☐   _____

# Hours Sleep	Bedtime	Wake Time	Sleep Quality
			😊 😐 😕 ☹️ ✖✖

Breakfast	Lunch	Dinner	Snacks

Notes: _____
_____
_____
_____
_____
_____
_____
_____
_____
_____

CELERY JUICE JOURNAL

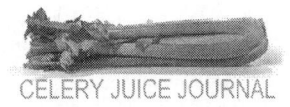

let the healing begin

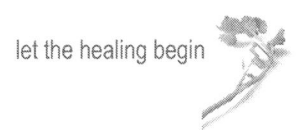

S M T W TH F S

Day # _____

Date: _____

Water: ☐☐☐☐☐
☐☐☐☐☐

Amount of Celery Juice: _____

Time of Celery Juice: _____

How I Feel Today: _____
_____

# Hours Sleep	Bedtime	Wake Time	Sleep Quality
			😊 🙂 😐 ☹️ 😵

Breakfast	Lunch	Dinner .	Snacks

Notes:
_____
_____
_____
_____
_____
_____
_____
_____
_____

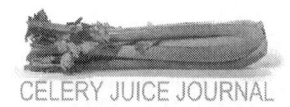

CELERY JUICE JOURNAL

let the healing begin

S M T W TH F S

Day # _____

Date: _____

Water: ☐☐☐☐☐
☐☐☐☐☐

Amount of Celery Juice: _____

Time of Celery Juice: _____

How I Feel Today: _____

# Hours Sleep	Bedtime	Wake Time	Sleep Quality
			😊 🙂 😐 ☹️ 😵

Breakfast	Lunch	Dinner .	Snacks

Notes: _____
_____
_____
_____
_____
_____
_____
_____
_____
_____

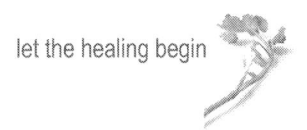

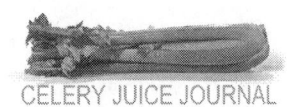

CELERY JUICE JOURNAL

let the healing begin

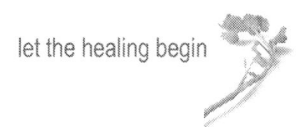

S M T W TH F S

Day # _____

Date: _____

Water: ☐☐☐☐☐
       ☐☐☐☐☐

Amount of Celery Juice: _____

Time of Celery Juice: _____

How I Feel Today: _____

# Hours Sleep	Bedtime	Wake Time	Sleep Quality
			😊 🙂 😐 ☹️ 😵

Breakfast	Lunch	Dinner	Snacks

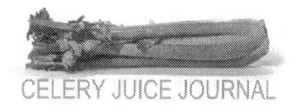

Notes:
_____
_____
_____
_____
_____
_____
_____
_____
_____
_____

CELERY JUICE JOURNAL

let the healing begin

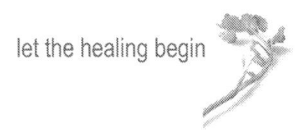

S M T W TH F S

Day # _____   Amount of Celery Juice: _____

Date: _____   Time of Celery Juice: _____

Water: ☐☐☐☐☐   How I Feel Today: _____
☐☐☐☐☐   _____

# Hours Sleep	Bedtime	Wake Time	Sleep Quality 😊 🙂 😐 🙁 😵

Breakfast	Lunch	Dinner .	Snacks

Notes: _____
_____
_____
_____
_____
_____
_____
_____
_____
_____
_____

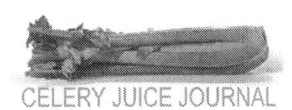

CELERY JUICE JOURNAL

let the healing begin

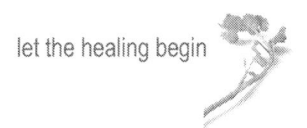

S M T W TH F S

Day # _____   Amount of Celery Juice: _____

Date: _____   Time of Celery Juice: _____

Water: ☐☐☐☐☐   How I Feel Today: _____
       ☐☐☐☐☐   _____

# Hours Sleep	Bedtime	Wake Time	Sleep Quality
			😊 🙂 😐 ☹️ 😣

Breakfast	Lunch	Dinner .	Snacks

Notes:
_____
_____
_____
_____
_____
_____
_____
_____
_____
_____

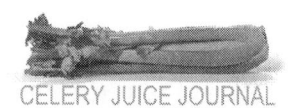

CELERY JUICE JOURNAL

let the healing begin

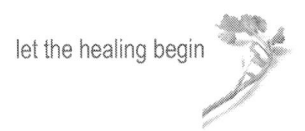

S M T W TH F S

Day # _____   Amount of Celery Juice: _____

Date: _____   Time of Celery Juice: _____

Water: ☐☐☐☐☐   How I Feel Today: _____
☐☐☐☐☐   _____

# Hours Sleep	Bedtime	Wake Time	Sleep Quality
			😊 🙂 😐 ☹️ 😵

Breakfast	Lunch	Dinner	Snacks

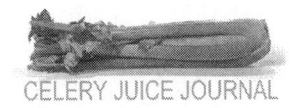

Notes: _____
_____
_____
_____
_____
_____
_____
_____
_____

CELERY JUICE JOURNAL

let the healing begin

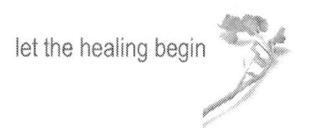

S M T W TH F S

Day # _____

Date: _____

Water: ☐☐☐☐☐
☐☐☐☐☐

Amount of Celery Juice: _____

Time of Celery Juice: _____

How I Feel Today: _____
_____

# Hours Sleep	Bedtime	Wake Time	Sleep Quality
			😊 🙂 😐 ☹️ 😵

Breakfast	Lunch	Dinner .	Snacks

Notes:
_____
_____
_____
_____
_____
_____
_____
_____
_____

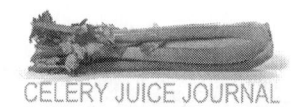

CELERY JUICE JOURNAL

let the healing begin

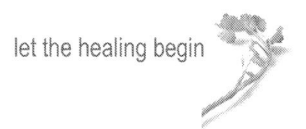

S M T W TH F S

Day # _____

Amount of Celery Juice: _____

Date: _____

Time of Celery Juice: _____

Water: ☐☐☐☐☐
☐☐☐☐☐

How I Feel Today: _____

_____

# Hours Sleep	Bedtime	Wake Time	Sleep Quality
			😊 🙂 😐 🙁 😵

Breakfast	Lunch	Dinner	Snacks

Notes:
_____
_____
_____
_____
_____
_____
_____
_____
_____
_____

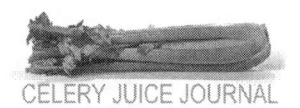

CELERY JUICE JOURNAL

let the healing begin

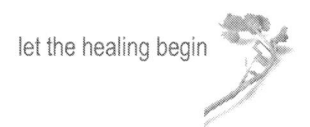

S M T W TH F S

Day # _____   Amount of Celery Juice: _____

Date: _____   Time of Celery Juice: _____

Water: ☐☐☐☐☐   How I Feel Today: _____
       ☐☐☐☐☐   _____

# Hours Sleep	Bedtime	Wake Time	Sleep Quality 😊 🙂 😐 ☹️ 😣

Breakfast	Lunch	Dinner	Snacks

Notes: _____
_____
_____
_____
_____
_____
_____
_____
_____

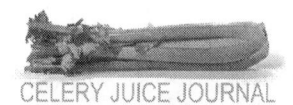

CELERY JUICE JOURNAL

let the healing begin

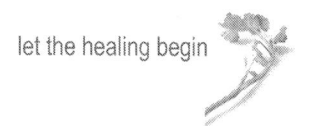

S   M   T   W   TH   F   S

Day # _____

Date: _____

Water: ☐☐☐☐☐
         ☐☐☐☐☐

Amount of Celery Juice: _____

Time of Celery Juice: _____

How I Feel Today: _____
_____

# Hours Sleep	Bedtime	Wake Time	Sleep Quality 😊 🙂 😐 🙁 😵

Breakfast	Lunch	Dinner .	Snacks

Notes:
_____
_____
_____
_____
_____
_____
_____
_____
_____
_____

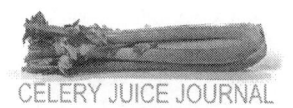

CELERY JUICE JOURNAL

let the healing begin

S   M   T   W   TH   F   S

Day # _____

Date: _____

Water: ☐☐☐☐☐
☐☐☐☐☐

Amount of Celery Juice: _____

Time of Celery Juice: _____

How I Feel Today: _____
_____

# Hours Sleep	Bedtime	Wake Time	Sleep Quality 😊 🙂 😐 ☹️ 😵

Breakfast	Lunch	Dinner .	Snacks

Notes:
_____
_____
_____
_____
_____
_____
_____
_____
_____

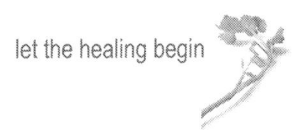

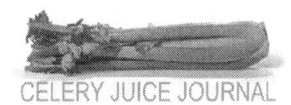

CELERY JUICE JOURNAL

let the healing begin

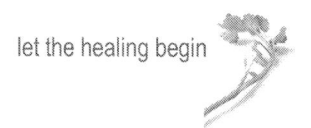

S M T W TH F S

Day # _____   Amount of Celery Juice: _____

Date: _____   Time of Celery Juice: _____

Water: ☐☐☐☐☐   How I Feel Today: _____
       ☐☐☐☐☐   _____

# Hours Sleep	Bedtime	Wake Time	Sleep Quality 😊 😐 😕 ☹ 😵

Breakfast	Lunch	Dinner	Snacks

Notes:
_____
_____
_____
_____
_____
_____
_____
_____
_____
_____
_____

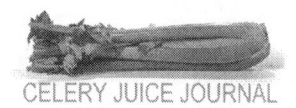

CELERY JUICE JOURNAL

let the healing begin

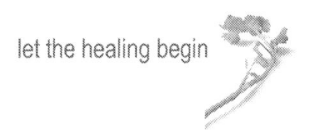

S   M   T   W   TH   F   S

Day # _____   Amount of Celery Juice: _____

Date: _____   Time of Celery Juice: _____

Water: ☐☐☐☐☐   How I Feel Today: _____
       ☐☐☐☐☐   _____

# Hours Sleep	Bedtime	Wake Time	Sleep Quality
			😊 😐 🙁 ☹ 😵

Breakfast	Lunch	Dinner .	Snacks

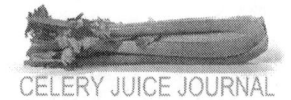

Notes:
_____
_____
_____
_____
_____
_____
_____
_____
_____
_____

CELERY JUICE JOURNAL

let the healing begin

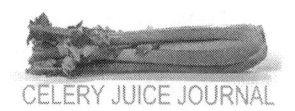

S M T W TH F S

Day # _____   Amount of Celery Juice: _____

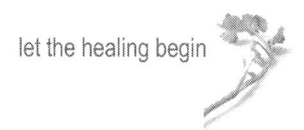

Date: _____   Time of Celery Juice: _____

Water: ☐☐☐☐☐   How I Feel Today: _____
       ☐☐☐☐☐   _____

# Hours Sleep	Bedtime	Wake Time	Sleep Quality
			😊 🙂 😐 🙁 😵

Breakfast	Lunch	Dinner	Snacks

Notes: _____
_____
_____
_____
_____
_____
_____
_____
_____
_____
_____

CELERY JUICE JOURNAL

let the healing begin

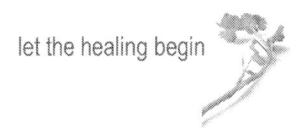

S M T W TH F S

Day # _____   Amount of Celery Juice: _____

Date: _____   Time of Celery Juice: _____

Water: ☐☐☐☐☐   How I Feel Today: _____
       ☐☐☐☐☐   _____

# Hours Sleep	Bedtime	Wake Time	Sleep Quality
			😊 🙂 😐 😕 😣

Breakfast	Lunch	Dinner .	Snacks

Notes:
_____
_____
_____
_____
_____
_____
_____
_____
_____
_____

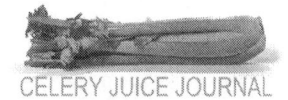

CELERY JUICE JOURNAL

let the healing begin

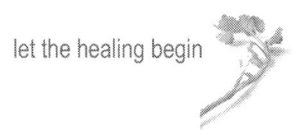

S M T W TH F S

Day # _____   Amount of Celery Juice: _____

Date: _____   Time of Celery Juice: _____

Water: ☐☐☐☐☐   How I Feel Today: _____
       ☐☐☐☐☐   _____

# Hours Sleep	Bedtime	Wake Time	Sleep Quality 😊 🙂 😐 🙁 😵

Breakfast	Lunch	Dinner .	Snacks

Notes: _____

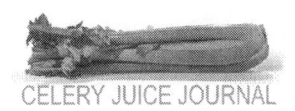

_____

_____

_____

_____

_____

_____

_____

_____

_____

CELERY JUICE JOURNAL

let the healing begin

S M T W TH F S

Day # _____   Amount of Celery Juice: _____

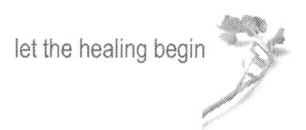

Date: _____   Time of Celery Juice: _____

Water: ☐☐☐☐☐   How I Feel Today: _____
       ☐☐☐☐☐   _____

# Hours Sleep	Bedtime	Wake Time	Sleep Quality
			😊 🙂 😐 🙁 😖

Breakfast	Lunch	Dinner .	Snacks

Notes:
_____
_____
_____
_____
_____
_____
_____
_____
_____

CELERY JUICE JOURNAL

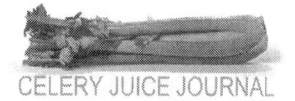

let the healing begin

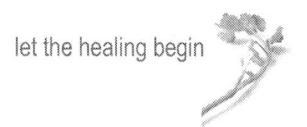

S M T W TH F S

Day #: _____

Date: _____

Water: ☐☐☐☐☐ ☐☐☐☐☐

Amount of Celery Juice: _____

Time of Celery Juice: _____

How I Feel Today: _____

# Hours Sleep	Bedtime	Wake Time	Sleep Quality
			😊 😐 😕 ☹️ ✖✖

Breakfast	Lunch	Dinner	Snacks

Notes:
_____
_____
_____
_____
_____
_____
_____
_____
_____
_____

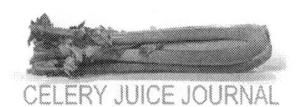

CELERY JUICE JOURNAL

let the healing begin

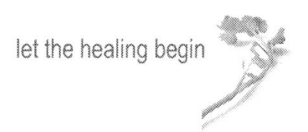

S M T W TH F S

Day # _____

Date: _____

Water: ☐☐☐☐☐
☐☐☐☐☐

Amount of Celery Juice: _____

Time of Celery Juice: _____

How I Feel Today: _____
_____

# Hours Sleep	Bedtime	Wake Time	Sleep Quality
			😊 🙂 😐 😟 😵

Breakfast	Lunch	Dinner .	Snacks

Notes:
_____
_____
_____
_____
_____
_____
_____
_____
_____
_____

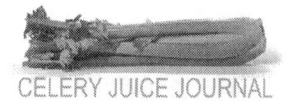

CELERY JUICE JOURNAL

let the healing begin

S M T W TH F S

Day # _____   Amount of Celery Juice: _____

Date: _____   Time of Celery Juice: _____

Water: ☐☐☐☐☐   How I Feel Today: _____
       ☐☐☐☐☐   _____

# Hours Sleep	Bedtime	Wake Time	Sleep Quality 😊 🙂 😐 🙁 😵

Breakfast	Lunch	Dinner	Snacks

Notes:
_____
_____
_____
_____
_____
_____
_____
_____
_____
_____

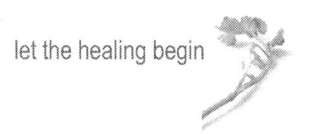

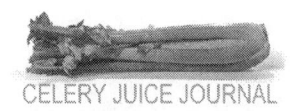

CELERY JUICE JOURNAL

let the healing begin

S M T W TH F S

Day # _____

Date: _____

Water: ☐☐☐☐☐
☐☐☐☐☐

Amount of Celery Juice: _____

Time of Celery Juice: _____

How I Feel Today: _____
_____

# Hours Sleep	Bedtime	Wake Time	Sleep Quality 😊 🙂 😐 😕 😣

Breakfast	Lunch	Dinner	Snacks

Notes:
_____
_____
_____
_____
_____
_____
_____
_____
_____

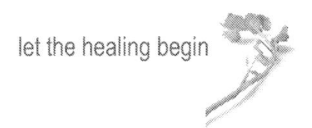

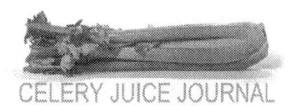

CELERY JUICE JOURNAL

let the healing begin

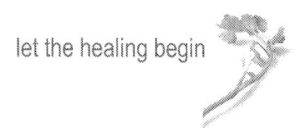

S   M   T   W   TH   F   S

Day # _____   Amount of Celery Juice: _____

Date: _____   Time of Celery Juice: _____

Water: ☐☐☐☐☐   How I Feel Today: _____
       ☐☐☐☐☐   _____

# Hours Sleep	Bedtime	Wake Time	Sleep Quality
			😊 😐 😕 ☹️ 😵

Breakfast	Lunch	Dinner	Snacks

Notes: _____
_____
_____
_____
_____
_____
_____
_____
_____
_____

CELERY JUICE JOURNAL

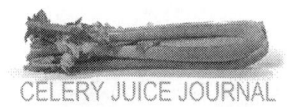

let the healing begin

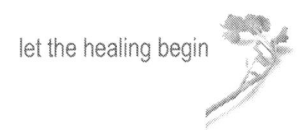

S M T W TH F S

Day # _____   Amount of Celery Juice: _____

Date: _____   Time of Celery Juice: _____

Water: ☐☐☐☐☐   How I Feel Today: _____
       ☐☐☐☐☐   _____

# Hours Sleep	Bedtime	Wake Time	Sleep Quality
			😊 🙂 😐 🙁 😫

Breakfast	Lunch	Dinner .	Snacks

Notes: _____

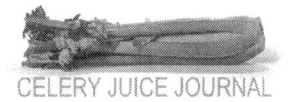

_____

_____

_____

_____

_____

_____

_____

_____

_____

CELERY JUICE JOURNAL

let the healing begin

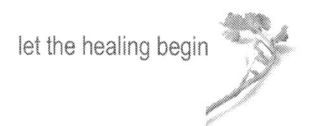

S M T W TH F S

Day # _____

Date: _____

Water: ☐☐☐☐☐ ☐☐☐☐☐

Amount of Celery Juice: _____

Time of Celery Juice: _____

How I Feel Today: _____

# Hours Sleep	Bedtime	Wake Time	Sleep Quality
			😊 😐 ☹ 😢 😵

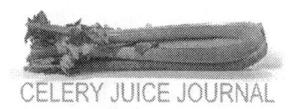

Breakfast	Lunch	Dinner	Snacks

Notes: _____
_____
_____
_____
_____
_____
_____
_____
_____

CELERY JUICE JOURNAL

let the healing begin

Notes

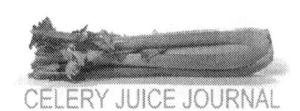

CELERY JUICE JOURNAL

let the healing begin

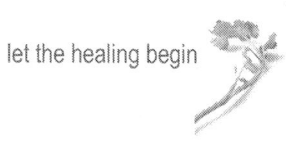

Notes

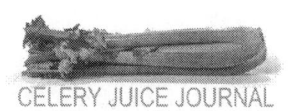

let the healing begin

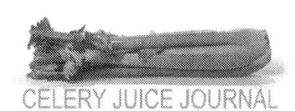

Notes

CELERY JUICE JOURNAL

let the healing begin

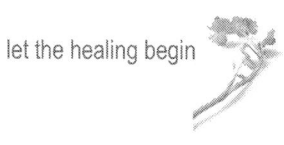

Notes

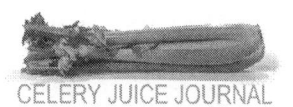

CELERY JUICE JOURNAL

let the healing begin

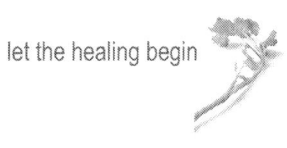

Notes

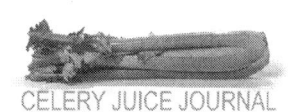

Manufactured by Amazon.ca
Bolton, ON